LITTLE BLUE PREVENTIVE MEDICINE SERIES: CANCER

Kwasi Yeboah-Afihene

Copyright © 2013 Kwasi Yeboah-Afihene

Library of Congress Control Number: 2013911065
ISBN-13: 978-1490317434
ISBN-10: 1490317430

This book was printed in the United States of America.

Publisher's contact details:

kwasi_afihene@yahoo.com

Dedication:

This book is dedicated to my Sister, Mrs. Eunice Donkor, who lost her battle with Ovarian Cancer in London General Hospital in 1999, and also to my Cousin, Nana Kofi Adom Boakye, and my two friends and mentors at UMDNJ - Rutgers University; Dr. Denish Mital and Dr. Shankar Srinivasan, and also a very good friend, Dr. Daniel Osei-Fofie, a radiation oncologist in South Africa, and cancer patients all over the world.

Acknowledgements

I am once again thankful to the Almighty for his grace, love, protection, and guidance for my life. I would like to express my profound gratitude to two very important personalities in my life: my father (now deceased) and my mother. Thanks to my dad for his love and confidence in me, and his wise counsel, and also to my mother, for the same, and introducing me to Christ. I would like to thank my children, Racquelle and Jeremiah for their love and patience.

Thanks to all my friends and family members for their confidence in me, and also for their help in such trying times. Another special thanks to the following people, who took time out of their very busy schedules to accept and review this work, most of all, to the brain children of all these wonderful ideas/inventions and the authors of the various articles from which they were extracted. Also much gratitude to the National Cancer Institute:

- ❖ Dr. William Ofori-Ntim, MD , Cardiologist, Wake Forest University Medical School, NC
- ❖ Dr. Joseph Osei, MD, Occupational Health – Entrepreneur, Dallas Texas
- ❖ Mr. Kwami Asiama, Accra Ghana / VA USA
- ❖ Dr. Yaw Ofori Abu, MD, Pulmonologist, Wellington FL
- ❖ Dr. Rebecca Abu, Pediatrician, MD, Wellington FL
- ❖ Dr. Kwaku Ampadu, PhD. Professor, Berkley College NJ/NY
- ❖ Mr. Okyere Bonna, Okab Publishing, Charlotte, NC

- ❖ Mr. Yaw Ofori Abu Jr. , Prospective Yale University Medical Student (Fall 2013)
- ❖ Dr. Isaac Kwaku Boamah, PhD. Author, Roselle NJ

Thank you all for your time and good work. I will finally apologize to all direct and indirect contributors I missed in my personal acknowledgements. Please forgive me, and accept my apologies, and most sincere gratitude for all your good work, which I believe will serve and help many lead healthy and quality lives.

PREFACE:

The efficacy of Cancer treatments are primarily base on medical diagnostic tests, and most of these are image driven. The images which results from the various tests, help medical practitioners in the field of Oncology properly identify tumors and their stages of progression. The results of the imaging process has to show enough details with clarity, to help determine how far the cancer has spread, (e.g. from tissues to lymph nodes .....) to enable proper staging of the Cancer. Improperly staged cancer, which compromises the appropriate severity of the symptoms and damages, usually warrants itself to the wrong therapeutic interventions, which often are not effective in treating the respective cancer tumors.

The question therefore is to investigate how medical image processing can effectively enhance the accuracy of cancer detection, diagnosis and treatment, using imaging techniques, with a special focus on molecular imaging. The content is presented in a very simple and easily comprehensible form.

The evidence as presented in this book, which are primarily ideas from numerous research work of others and inferences drawn from them, clearly shows the immense critical role medical imaging plays in the diagnosis, staging, and management of various forms of cancer. It also highlights the role Molecular imaging specifically, play in improving clinical understanding of various tumors, and decision making on their cure or treatment.

The second part of the material provides general insights to cancer management and prevention. It does so, in an effort to provide information to interested parties, enhancing their understanding of the illness, its preventive measures, and management strategies. It is mostly geared towards patients and people at risk with little or no healthcare experience.

My role in this book was primarily reviewing, summarizing, and integrating ideas from numerous research work, text books and other medical journals. I must humbly submit that, these are not my personal ideas or findings. Besides some inferences drawn and some personal analysis done, they are all borrowed ideas which I put together in a more centralized and coherent form, to give desperate and anxious patients a good start. This I believe will go a long way to help unnerve their anxieties from lack of knowledge about their diagnosis and prognosis, as well as what to expect down the road.

It highlights particularly, how critical medical and molecular imaging is, to the field of oncology, and cancer diagnosis and management specifically. And also how to mitigate the risk of the disease's incident by being aware of major risk factors, and making adjustments to one's lifestyle, to avert the otherwise apparent misfortune. Its casual and simplicity in writing style was intentional. The idea was to accommodate the wide spectrum of potential readers, who may span varying levels of literary competencies.

This book is by no means a replacement for proper expert consultation and advice from a trained and experienced doctor. It is a piece of information to improve patients' understanding of the disease and its management, and hopefully increase awareness of preventive measures. It will also help them in having an intelligent and informed conversation with their health care professionals. The granularity of the Table of Content is to help patient move to specific topics of interest with ease. It may look like an over kill, but I believe it will rather be a saving grace for some, who may be under pressure to find a specific information.

LITTLE BLUE PEVENTIVE MEDICIN SERIES: CANCER

By

Kwasi Yeboah-Afihene

This is very insightful information on Cancer, and is tailored towards helping both patients and people at risk for getting cancer, gather invaluable educational information on the disease. It is however not a replacement for medical consultation with a certified professional. Some healthcare workers in the field of oncology may also find it very useful.

Table of Contents:

XIX

INTRODUCTION:

In December 1999, I called my sister in London to find out how she and family were doing. To my surprise and dismay, the news was broken to me by my brother in-law that she has been admitted to the hospital with cancer. I was very stunned and confused. I quickly asked how she was doing. Quite well, my brother in law said.

I got her phone number, and called her at the hospital. She sounded very pleasant, and that gave me an assurance that she is in good spirits. I managed to quickly make arrangements to visit her in London. I spent Christmas with them and return shortly after that.

Upon my returned, I call home to inform my Dad that I have seen Eunice, and she is in very good spirits. Before I ended my first sentence, my Dad interjected, and asked if I have heard from my Brother in-law. I said no. He sobbed for a moment, and broke the news to me that she could not make it, and passed away shortly after I left London. This really did break my heart, and l lapsed into an immense sorrow. God and time was my only source of consolation.

During my career at AT&T Cooperation, I met a wonderful Jewish gentleman call Dr. Howard Alex, a very nice fellow, with a chemical engineering background. After collaborating with him in a couple of projects, we became friends.

In other not to recount another sad story to stair your emotions in a negative way, I will cut his story short. Howard also lost two successive wives to cancer, one of whom I became very well acquainted with, due to my frequency to their home upon invitations, in Marlboro New Jersey.

Cancer has become too close to call for me. Needless to say, another very dear cousin and the wife of another very good friend, also became victims. The good part in these gloomy successive cancer episodes is that, they both survived, and are now living a very good quality life.

Preventive medicine is broad, and I believe preventing obesity should have taken the central stage, and be the first topic to discus in this series. However I chose cancer because of it deadly nature, and the uncertainties still hovering around its cause and management.

This book explores the role of medical imaging in oncology, especially in the area of cancer detection, diagnosis, treatment, and also its prevention. It especially highlights amongst others, the recent advances in medical imaging, pertaining to the molecular imaging area. Advancement in imaging technologies, and related tracers, has greatly facilitated the identification and quantization of biomarkers. It has unleashed a lot of insights in the cellular and molecular genesis of Cancer. This has greatly improved the detection, maintenance and treatment of the disease. Although the clinical interpretations of biomarkers are of interdisciplinary dimensions, the focus is going to be on medical and molecular imaging.

A general insight into oncology, cancer detection and treatment options, will be shared to enhance the readers understanding of the entire cancer treatment and management process. It is by no means exhaustive of the myriad of information out there. It is however a very good start.

EXAMPLES OF IMAGING APPLICATIONS IN MEDICINE AND BIO-MEDICAL RESEARCH:

The diversity of image processing applications, and their universality, and versatility across many functional disciplines and industries, make it a very powerful and important topic to be familiar with.. The need to understand its basics is quite close to learning "ABC" in the good old tender ages, around the onset of our academic, and career pursuits. I cannot exhaust the extensive usage of image processing in today world in this book; however these are a few applications worth noting.

Biological and biomedical Research; The analysis of components of biological samples which can sometimes be automated by digital imaging:

- ✓ Image enhancement – Techniques for improving the visibility of features that are not evident in the original image, such as contrast balancing and edge sharpening.
- ✓ Bone, tissue and cell analysis – automatic counting and classification of cell structures and other objects.
- ✓ DNA typing – analysis, classification and matching of DNA material

Medical Diagnostic Imaging:

The impacts of medical diagnostic imaging in medicine have really advanced the evidence based medicine paradigm, and have elevate it to a different level. It has enabled many advanced therapeutic interventions to be administered to patients, which precisely target respective indications and help cure or manage symptoms for patients', improving their quality of life. Medical and radiological imaging looks at the internal components of the human body, and help in the precise diagnosis and treatment of many medical indications including cancer and others. The following are a few areas of interest:

- ✓ Image enhancements
- ✓ Digital subtraction angiography
- ✓ Computed tomography
- ✓ PET

Modern
Superconducting MRI
System

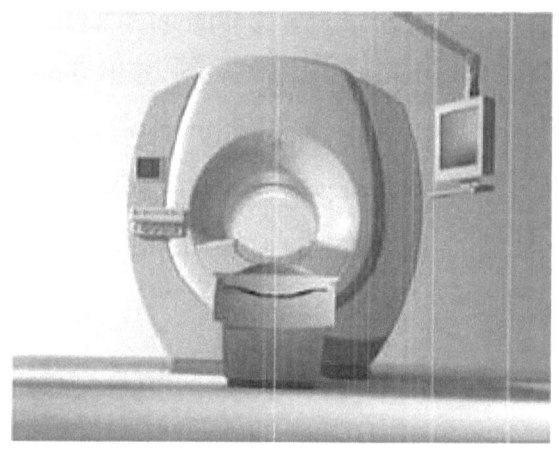

Courtesy of: Philips Corporation.

Schema of a PET acquisition process

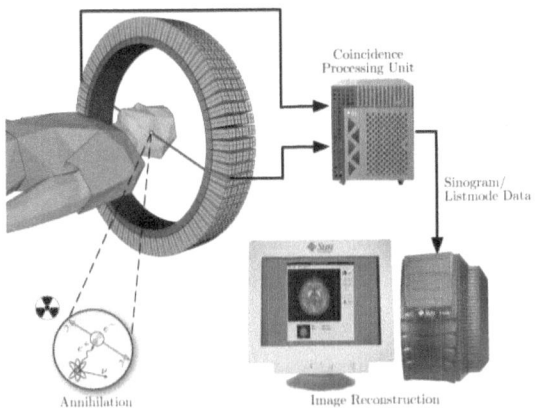

PET Schema – Wikipedia:
(http://www.wikipedia.org)

ONCOLOGY

According to the medical-dictionary.thefeedictionary.com, oncology is the branch of medicine, dealing with the physical, chemical, and biological properties of tumors, including study of their development, diagnosis, treatment and prevention.

> ➤ The study of tumors
> ➤ Totality of medical knowledge concerning tumors

It can also be viewed as the branch of medicine, concerned with the study, classification, and treatment of tumor. Cancer however is one of the major forms of deadly tumors categorized under the domain of oncology. The rest of this book will be primarily concerned with Oncology with respect to cancer diagnosis prevention and management, using medical imaging techniques and others.

VARIOUS FORMS OF CANCER

The following is a list of a few forms of Cancer, though not exhaustive of the entire types known. There are several forms of cancer tumors, which span a spectrum of aggressive to benign types. The aggressiveness of the tumor characterizes the rate at which it spreads to other tissues and organs whiles the latter expresses its dormancy or non threatening state.

No one can exhaustively cover all of them in detail with enough depth effectively in one book. Else it will be a very big volume. We will therefore talk about a few. *(The list's source: The National Cancer Institute; www.caner.gov)*

A

Acute Lymphoblastic Leukemia (ALL)
Acute Myeloid Leukemia (AML)
Adolescents, Cancer in
Adrenocortical Carcinoma
    Childhood
AIDS-Related Cancers
    Kaposi Sarcoma
    Lymphoma
Anal Cancer

Appendix Cancer

Astrocytomas, Childhood

    Atypical Teratoid/Rhabdoid Tumor,

Childhood, Central Nervous System

B

Basal Cell Carcinoma - see Skin Cancer

(Nonmelanoma)

Bile Duct Cancer, Extrahepatic

Bladder Cancer

    Childhood

Bone Cancer, Osteosarcoma and Malignant

Fibrous Histiocytoma

Brain Stem Glioma, Childhood

Brain Tumor

    Astrocytomas, Childhood

    Brain and Spinal Cord Tumors,

Childhood

    Brain Stem Glioma, Childhood

    Central Nervous System Atypical

14

Teratoid/Rhabdoid Tumor, Childhood
Central Nervous System Embryonal
Tumors, Childhood
Central Nervous System Germ Cell
Tumors, Childhood
Craniopharyngioma, Childhood
Ependymoblastoma, Childhood
Ependymoma, Childhood
Medulloblastoma, Childhood
Medulloepithelioma,
Childhood
Pineal Parenchymal Tumors of
Intermediate Differentiation,
Childhood
Supratentorial Primitive
Neuroectodermal Tumors and
Pineoblastoma, Childhood
Breast Cancer
Childhood
Male

Pregnancy, Breast Cancer and
Bronchial Tumors, Childhood
Burkitt Lymphoma - see Non-Hodgkin
Lymphoma

SUMMARY OF RISK FACTORS

Most of the ideas in this section and others were borrowed from the National Cancer Institute website *(www.cancer.gov)* and other listed sources.

Doctors often cannot explain why one person develops cancer and another does not. But research shows that certain risk factors increase the chance that a person will develop cancer. These are the most common risk factors for cancer of which illustrations and explanations will be provided later in the book:

- ➢ Growing older

- ➢ Tobacco

- ➢ Sunlight

- ➢ Ionizing radiation

- ➢ Certain chemicals and other substances

- ➢ Some viruses and bacteria

- ➢ Certain hormones

- ➢ Family history of cancer

- ➢ Alcohol

- ➢ Poor diet, lack of physical activity, or being overweight

Screening

Some types of cancer can be found before they cause symptoms. Checking for cancer (or for conditions that may lead to cancer) in people who have no symptoms is called screening. Screening can help doctors find and treat some types of cancer early. Generally, cancer treatment is more effective when the disease is found early. It is however very interesting to note that, most effective screening techniques, such as mammography uses medical imaging systems and processing techniques. This goes to highlight our initial point about the critical role imaging technologies and processing techniques play in the diagnosis and management of various forms of cancer. Screening tests are used widely to check for cancers of the breast, cervix, colon, and rectum:

➢ **Breast:** A mammogram

➢ **Cervix:** The Pap test (sometimes called Pap smear)

➤ **Colon and rectum:** A number of screening tests are used to detect polyps (growths), cancer, or other problems in the colon and rectum.

- Fecal occult blood test:

- Sigmoidoscopy:

- Colonoscopy:

- Double-contrast barium emena:

- Digital rectal exam

Symptoms

Cancer can cause many different symptoms. These are some of them:

A thickening or lump in the breast or any other part of the body

A new mole or a change in an existing mole

> A sore that does not heal

> Hoarseness or a cough that does not go away

> Changes in bowel or bladder habits

> Discomfort after eating

> A hard time swallowing

> Weight gain or loss with no known reason

> Unusual bleeding or discharge

> Feeling weak or very tired

Most often, these symptoms are not due to only cancer. They may also be caused by benign tumors or other problems. Only a doctor can tell for sure. Anyone with these symptoms or other changes in health should see a doctor to diagnose and treat problems as early as possible.

SOCIO – ECONOMIC EFFECT OF CANCER

Cancer has an insurmountable and gruesome effect in many different dimensions. It affects patient very adversely due to its incapacitating and painful nature, as well as negative financial impact to the family. The high cost of treatment of cancer can eat into one's lifetime nest egg, if the appropriate insurance policies are not in place to help manage the risk. Inability to lead a much more active lifestyle, can also leads to poor productivity, and hence loss of income potential depending on the severity of it.

The other dimension worth noting is the effect on the family. Cancer takes a big toll on the nuclear family's financial and emotional health,in such a way that, the future of the entire members becomes crippled, due to lack of money. The healthy Spouses are put under a tremendous pressure, financially and emotionally to sustain the family. This sometimes, depending on the lifetime earning potential of the unhealthy spouse, could almost be impossible for the family to survive, and potentially slip them into extreme poverty.

Depending on the age of the patient, it can also have a big toll on the extended family as well. Seeking and arranging custodial help for parents with cancer could also spin the children in a spiral mode of stress and confusion, hence distracting their respective family balance.

For businesses, the loss of productivity and skills cannot be emphasized enough. The financial and economic toll on the country in general is so huge, due to obvious cost ripples. Lots of money goes into cancer research, while a lot more goes into its diagnosis, and management. The death toll due to cancer however has improved over the years, yet it is still among the leaders.

Diagnosis

If you have a symptom, or your screening test result suggests cancer, the doctor must find out whether it is due to cancer or to some other causes. Family medical history, physical exam, and a couple of lab and imaging tests including Molecular imaging techniques, help doctors to confirm their suspicions finally with a biopsy.

Lab Tests

Tests of the blood, urine, or other fluids can help doctors make a diagnosis. These tests can show how well an organ (such as the kidney) is doing its job.

Imaging Procedures

Imaging procedures create pictures of areas inside your body that help the doctor see whether a tumor is present. It is also worth noting here that, without these images, produced by using the under listed technologies, it would have been very difficult to impossible , for practitioners to have an understanding of the nature of the tumor they are dealing with, let alone know where it is, to even operate on it, if it requires surgery. These pictures can be made in several ways:

> **X-rays:**

> **CT Scan:**

> **Radionuclide scan:**

> **Ultrasound: MRI:**

26

➢ **PET Scan:**

Biopsy

For a biopsy, the doctor removes a sample of tissue and sends it to a lab. A pathologist looks at the tissue under a microscope. The sample may be removed in several ways:

➢ **With a needle:** The doctor uses a needle to withdraw tissue or fluid.

➢ **With an endoscope:** The doctor uses a thin, lighted tube (an endoscope) to look at areas inside the body. The doctor can remove tissue or cells through the tube.

➢ **With surgery:** Surgery may be excision or incision.

- In an excision biopsy, the surgeon removes the entire tumor. Often some of the normal tissue around the tumor also is removed.

- In an incision biopsy, the surgeon removes just part of the tumor.

Staging

To plan the best treatment for cancer, the doctor needs to know the extent (Stage) of your disease. For most cancers (such as breast, lung, prostate, or colon cancer), the stage is based on the size of the tumor and whether the cancer has spread to lymph nodes or other parts of the body.

Treatment

Many people with cancer want to take an active part in making decisions about their medical care. It is natural to want to learn all you can about your disease and treatment choices. However, shock and stress after the diagnosis can make it hard to think of everything you want to ask the doctor. It often helps to make a list of questions before an appointment.

To help remember what the doctor says, you may take notes or ask whether you may use a tape recorder. Some people also want to have a family member or friend with them when they talk to the doctor - to take part in the discussion, to take notes, or just to listen.

You do not need to ask all your questions at once. You will have other chances to ask the doctor or nurse to explain things that are not clear and to ask for more information.

Your doctor may refer you to a specialist, or you may ask for a referral. Specialists who treat cancer include surgeons, medical oncologists, hematologist, and radiation oncologists.

Getting a Second Opinion

Before starting treatment, you may want a second opinion about your diagnosis and treatment plan. Many insurance companies will cover a second opinion if your doctor requests it. It may take some time and effort to gather medical records and arrange to see another doctor. Usually it is not a problem to take several weeks to get a second opinion.

In most cases, the delay in starting treatment will not make treatment less effective. But some people with cancer need treatment right away. To make sure, you should discuss this delay with your doctor.

Treatment Methods

The treatment plan depends mainly on the type of cancer and the stage of the disease both of which are catalyzed by imaging technologies and processing techniques. These highlights about imaging at various sections of this book, is just to help buttress our initial accessions. Doctors also consider the patient's age and general health. Often, the goal of treatment is to cure the cancer. In other cases, the goal is to control the disease or to reduce symptoms for as long as possible. The treatment plan may change over time.

Most treatment plans include surgery, radiation therapy, or chemotherapy. Some involve hormone therapy or biological therapy. In addition, stem cell transplantation may be used so that a patient can receive very high doses of chemotherapy or radiation therapy.

Some cancers respond best to a single type of treatment. Others may respond best to a combination of treatments.

Treatments may work in a specific area (local therapy) or throughout the body (systemic therapy):

> **Local therapy** removes or destroys cancer in just one part of the body.

Surgery to remove a tumor is local therapy. Radiation to shrink or destroy a tumor also is usually local therapy.

➤ **Systemic therapy** sends drugs or substances through the bloodstream to destroy cancer cells all over the body. It kills or slows the growth of cancer cells that may have spread beyond the original tumor. Chemotherapy, hormone therapy, and biological therapy are usually systemic therapy.

Complementary and Alternative Medicine

Some people with cancer use complementary and alternative medicine (CAM):

> ➢ An approach is generally called complementary medicine when it is used along with standard treatment.

> ➢ An approach is called alternative medicine when it is used instead of standard treatment.

Nutrition and Physical Activity

It is important for people with cancer to take care of themselves. Taking care of yourself includes eating well and staying as active as you can. You need enough calories to maintain a good weight. You also need enough protein to keep up your strength. Eating well may help you feel better and have more energy.

Many people find they feel better when they stay active. Walking, yoga, swimming, and other activities can keep you strong and increase your energy. Exercise may reduce nausea and pain and make treatment easier to handle. It also can help relieve stress.

Follow-up Care

Advances in early detection and treatment make it possible for many people with cancer to be cured. But doctors can never be certain that the cancer will not come back.

Undetected, cancer cells can remain in the body after treatment. Although the cancer seems to be completely removed or destroyed, it can return. Doctors call this a recurrence.

CANCER STAGING AND THE ROLE OF MEDICAL IMAGING

Cancer may be difficult to detect, but for some types of cancer, the earlier it is detected, the better are the chances of treating it effectively. Imaging techniques - methods of producing pictures of the body - have become an important element of early detection for many cancers. But imaging is not simply used for detection. Imaging is also important for determining the stage (telling how advanced the cancer is) and the precise locations of cancer to aid in directing surgery and other cancer treatments, or to check if a cancer has returned.

Clinical trials, research studies involving people, play an essential role in determining whether emerging imaging techniques are effective and safe.

MOLECULAR IMAGING AND ONCOLOGY:

As per the article, "Recent advances in molecular imaging and biomarkers in cancer…" published in Drug Discovery Today, "Molecular imaging is the visualization, characterization and measurement of biological processes at the molecular and cellular level. In oncology, molecular imaging approaches can be directly, applied as translational biomarkers of disease progression…."

A.

Current role of imaging in cancer management:

An example: Advance Lung Analysis Lesion Sizing from 3D CT:

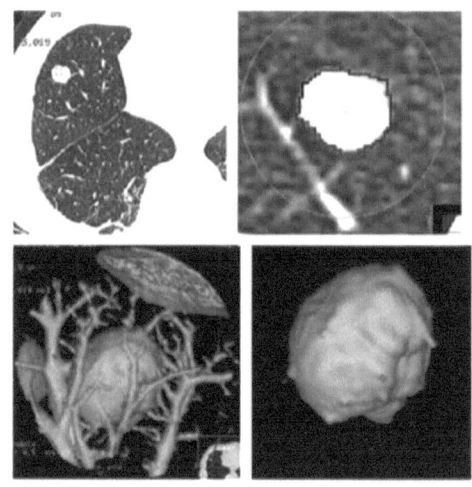

BRIEF LITERATURE REVIEWS

This section of the book is going to highlight research finding in the role imaging (Molecular Imaging) play or is going to play in the future, in the diagnosis and management of cancer. It is going to be in the form of highlights and conclusions about the various articles with illustrative images to clarify the point if necessary. Several articles were reviewed but will only present a few that are representative of the ideas that are being emphasized in this book.

I.   Sohaib et al.

"Diagnosis, Staging, and Management of Testicular Cancers."

As per the research findings, most people with testicular GCTs can now be expected to be cured, ones an appropriate management strategy is in place. Central to this management strategy is medical imaging technologies such as MRI, CT and PET. CT. These remain the core imaging technology central to the selection of good management strategy to cure the disease. In order to avoid systemic toxicity and other possible long term complications, medical imaging helps to target the tumors more precisely. The potential of MRI and PET continue to evolve with a lot of promise in this area according to their findings. These are a few examples of images, showing how the related technologies are used to Diagnose, Stage and manage testicular cancer:

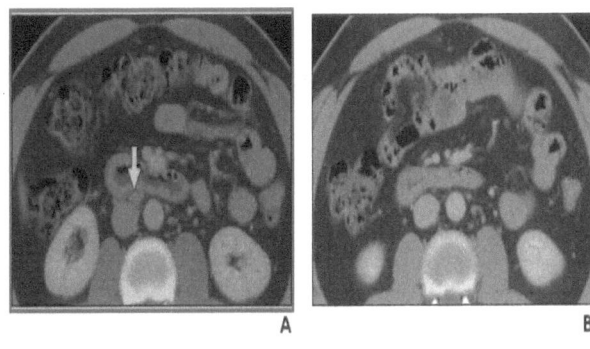

42-year-old man with stage IIA disease from right-sided nonseminomatous germ cell tumor. Contrastenhanced CT shows response to chemotherapy.

A, CT scan shows 10-mm aortocaval node (*arrow*) behind third part of duodenum.

B, CT scan obtained after patient underwent treatment with chemotherapy shows that there has been complete response.

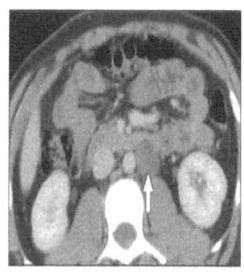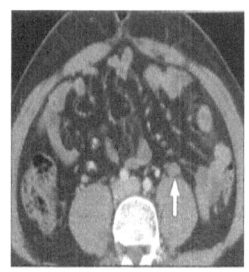

23-year-old man with stage IIB disease

From left-sided nonseminomatous germ cell tumor.

Contrast-enhanced CT scan shows 4-cm left

Par aortic node (*arrow*).

24-year-old man with recurrent

Nonseminomatous germ cell tumor. Contrast enhanced

CT scan shows 1.5-cm echelon node

(*Arrow*) on left psoas muscle.

II.   Elsevier. et al
Imaging and cancer: A review:

Different types of biomedical imaging techniques together are used in all phases of cancer management. Medical imaging is critically essential in cancer clinical protocols and is able to furnish morphological, structural, metabolic and functional

44

information. Together with other diagnostic tools, (e.g. in vitro tissue and fluids analysis) assists in clinical decision-making. Hybrid imaging techniques are also able to supply information for improved staging and therapy planning. Targeted minimally invasive therapy guided by medical imaging, has the promise to improve outcome and reduce collateral effects.

Early detection of cancer through screening based on imaging is one of the major contributors to a reduction in mortality for certain cancers. Medical imaging is therefore very pivotal in all phases of cancer management and without it, targeted therapeutic interventions would have been almost extinct and systemic toxicity of patients due to contamination of healthy cells with strong and sometime toxic chemicals and radiation would have been a common place. This would have eventually affected patient quality of life which could affect their emotional health and immune system in general.

Molecular imaging has made immense inroads in the management of cancer. The ability to detect real changes at the cellular and molecular level helps to target metastatic cell directly and apply appropriate interventions in the general area where the cancerous cells are present, therefore avoiding possible adverse effect on healthy neighboring cell.

III. Recent advances in molecular imaging biomarkers in cancer application of Bench to bedside technologies

An important direction of oncology research has been to develop new tumor-targeted therapies and diagnostic approaches for the early detection of malignancies. An important component in these activities has been the discovery and validation of new oncology biomarkers. The Biomarkers Definitions Workgroup, sponsored by the National Institutes of Health, stated in 2001 that 'a biological marker – biomarker – is a characteristic that is objectively measured and evaluated as an indicator of normal biological processes, pathogenic processes, or pharmacologic responses to a therapeutic intervention'. Currently, clinical size measurements of tumor lesions by computed tomography (CT) and magnetic resonance imaging (MRI) are the predominant ways in which disease progression and therapeutic drug efficacy are assessed. At the moment, the overall response and progression free survival are the only imaging biomarkers used as surrogate end-points to measure the effect of chemotherapy and radiation therapy in clinical trials according to the article.

Molecular imaging (MI) enables non-invasive monitoring of cellular processes at the molecular or genetic level, in vivo. MI modalities then can be used directly in oncology as biomarkers of disease progression. Also effects of new targeted anti-cancer therapies on cellular pathways and gene expression can also be monitored. Advances in imaging hardware and contrast agents or tracer, have resulted in the increasing role for MI in tumor diagnosis, monitoring tumor progression and the assessment of therapeutic effect. Tissue based or ex vivo imaging has also emerged as an important tool in the discovery and validation of oncology biomarkers in preclinical research.

Molecular imaging technologies used in detecting biomarkers for monitor disease progression:

- ➤ Optical imaging: bioluminescence and fluorescence
- ➤ PET imaging
- ➤ SPECT Imaging

Molecular imaging technologies use for Tumor Metabolism:

- ➤ FDG PET
- ➤ MET PET
- ➤ FET PET
- ➤ FLT PET
- ➤ FDG PET
- ➤ C-ACETATE PET

Molecular imaging technologies used for Tumor Hypoxia:

- ➤ Cu-ATSM PET
- ➤ FMISO PET

Molecular imaging technologies used for Tumor receptor expression:

- ➢ FDG PET
- ➢ RGD PET
- ➢ DCE MRI

Multimodality Imaging:

By combining MI modalities, additive information can be used to further assess disease progression when compared with the use of a single imaging modality alone. The combination of several imaging modalities, such as PET/CT and SPECT/CT, to assess disease progression is widely used. The set back to this approach at the moment is that the images are taken sequentially and get combined with software.

Tissue-Based imaging in oncology biomarker discovery and validation:

Mass spectrometry-based imaging and infrared spectroscopy of tissues have emerged as two highly innovative approaches that provide key information regarding the misdistribution of molecules of interest (e.g. proteins, lipids) without the requirement of prior labeling. There is however a lot of work to be done to ensure its routine clinical use to sub classify human tumor tissues and predict patient outcome. However, automated image analysis approaches to advance histopathological recognition and quantization of biomarkers have gained considerable traction recently.

CONCLUSION:

Insight gained in the molecular genesis of cancer, as well as the increasing superiority of imaging technology, has helped translational researchers and clinicians in disease progressing monitoring, thus enabling patients to engage in preventive and or disease-retarding treatment regimens. The process of biomarker clinical translation is both complex and time consuming. Multiple and diverse technologies play a very important role in helping clinicians analyze and make the right decisions. Molecular imaging techniques and strategies amongst which is tissue based imaging have greatly facilitated important clinical and preliminary advances in the field of biomarker clinical translation and quantization.

SECTION II A: Rick factors Explained.

Major Risk Factors

These are the most common risk factors for cancer:

- Growing older

- Tobacco

- Sunlight

- Ionizing radiation

- Certain chemicals and other substances

- Some viruses and bacteria

- Certain Hormones

- Family history of cancer

- Alcohol

- Poor diet, lack of physical activity, or being overweight

Many of these risk factors can be avoided. Others, such as family history, cannot be avoided. People can help protect themselves by staying away from known risk factors whenever possible.

If you think you may be at risk for cancer, you should discuss this concern with your doctor. You may want to ask about reducing your risk and about a schedule for checkups.

Over time, several factors may act together to cause normal cells to become cancerous. When thinking about your risk of getting cancer, these are some things to keep in mind:

- Not everything causes cancer.

- Cancer is not caused by an injury, such as a bump or bruise.

- Cancer is not contagious. Although being infected with certain viruses or bacteria may increase the risk of some types of cancer, no one can "catch" cancer from another person.

- Having one or more risk factors does not mean that you will get cancer. Most people who have risk factors never develop cancer.

- Some people are more sensitive than others to the known risk factors.

The sections below have more detailed information about the most common risk factors for cancer.

Growing Older

The most important risk factor for cancer is growing older. Most cancers occur in people over the age of 65. But people of all ages, including children, can get cancer, too.

Tobacco

Tobacco use is the most preventable cause of death. Each year, more than 180,000 Americans die from cancer that is related to tobacco use.

Using tobacco products or regularly being around tobacco smoke (environmental or secondhand smoke) increases the risk of cancer.

Smokers are more likely than nonsmokers to develop cancer of the lung, larynx (voice box), mouth, esophagus, bladder, kidney, throat, stomach, pancreas, or cervix. They also are more likely to develop acute myeloid leukemia (cancer that starts in blood cells).

People who use smokeless tobacco (snuff or chewing tobacco) are at increased risk of cancer of the mouth.

Quitting is important for anyone who uses tobacco - even people who have used it for many years. The risk of cancer for people who quit is lower than the risk for people who continue to use tobacco. (But the risk of cancer is generally lowest among those who never used tobacco.)

Also, for people who have already had cancer, quitting may reduce the chance of getting another cancer.

There are many resources to help people stop using tobacco:

- Staff at the NCI's Smoking Quit line (1-877-44U-QUIT) and at **Live Help (http://www.cancer.gov/livehelp)** can talk with you about ways to quit smoking and about groups that help smokers who want to quit. Groups may offer counseling in person or by telephone.

- A Federal Government Web site, http://www.smokefree.gov, has an online guide to quitting smoking and a list of other resources.

- Doctors and dentists can help their patients find local programs or trained professionals who help people stop using tobacco.

- Doctors and dentists can suggest medicine or nicotine replacement therapy, such as a patch, gum, lozenge, nasal spray, or inhaler.

Sunlight

Ultraviolet (UV) radiation comes from the sun, sunlamps, and tanning booths. It causes early aging of the skin and skin damage that can lead to skin cancer.

Doctors encourage people of all ages to limit their time in the sun and to avoid other sources of UV radiation:

- It is best to avoid the midday sun (from mid-morning to late afternoon) whenever possible. You also should protect yourself from UV radiation reflected by sand, water, snow, and ice. UV radiation can penetrate light clothing, windshields, and windows.

- Wear long sleeves, long pants, a hat with a wide brim, and sunglasses with lenses that absorb UV.

- Use sunscreen. Sunscreen may help prevent skin cancer, especially sunscreen with a sun protection factor (SPF) of at least 15. But sunscreens cannot replace avoiding the sun and wearing clothing to protect the skin.

- Stay away from sunlamps and tanning booths. They are no safer than sunlight.

Protect yourself from the sun.

Ionizing Radiation

Ionizing radiation can cause cell damage that leads to cancer. This kind of radiation comes from rays that enter the Earth's atmosphere from outer space, radioactive fallout, radon gas, x-rays, and other sources.

Radioactive fallout can come from accidents at nuclear power plants or from the production, testing, or use of atomic weapons. People exposed to fallout may have an increased risk of cancer, especially leukemia and cancers of the thyroid, breast, lung, and stomach.

Radon is a radioactive gas that you cannot see, smell, or taste. It forms in soil and rocks. People who work in mines may be exposed to radon. In some parts of the country, radon is found in houses. People exposed to radon are at increased risk of lung cancer.

Medical procedures are a common source of radiation:

- Doctors use radiation (low-dose x-rays) to take pictures of the inside of the body. These pictures help to diagnose broken bones and other problems.

- Doctors use **radiation therapy** (high-dose radiation from large machines or from radioactive substances) to treat cancer.

The risk of cancer from low-dose x-rays is extremely small. The risk from radiation therapy is slightly higher. For both, the benefit nearly always outweighs the small risk.

You should talk with your doctor if you are concerned that you may be at risk for cancer due to radiation.

If you live in a part of the country that has radon, you may wish to test your home for high levels of the gas. The home radon test is easy to use and inexpensive. Most hardware stores sell the test kit.

You should talk with your doctor or dentist about the need for each x-ray. You should also ask about shields to protect parts of the body that are not in the picture.

Cancer patients may want to talk with their doctor about how radiation treatment could increase their risk of a second cancer later on.

Certain Chemicals and Other Substances

People who have certain jobs (such as painters, construction workers, and those in the chemical industry) have an increased risk of cancer. Many studies have shown that exposure to asbestos, benzene, Benzedrine, cadmium, nickel, or vinyl chloride in the workplace can cause cancer.

Follow instructions and safety tips to avoid or reduce contact with harmful substances both at work and at home. Although the risk is highest for workers with years of exposure, it makes sense to be careful at home when handling pesticides, used engine oil, paint, solvents, and other chemicals.

Some Viruses and Bacteria

Being infected with certain viruses or bacteria may increase the risk of developing cancer:

- Human Papillomaviruses (HPVs): HPV infection is the main cause of cervical cancer. It also may be a risk factor for other types of cancer.

- Hepatitis B and Hepatitis C viruses: Liver cancer can develop after many years of infection with hepatitis B or hepatitis C.

- Human T-Cell Leukemia virus (HTLV-1): Infection with HTLV-1 increases a person's risk of lymphoma and leukemia.

- Human immunodeficiency virus (HIV): HIV is the virus that causes AIDS. People who have HIV infection are at greater risk of cancer, such as lymphoma and a rare cancer called Kaposi.

- Epstein-Barr virus (EBV): Infection with EBV has been linked to an increased risk of lymphoma.

- Human Herpesvirus 8 (HHV8): This virus is a risk factor for Kaposi's sarcoma.

- Helicobacter pylori: This bacterium can cause stomach ulcers. It also can cause stomach cancer and lymphoma in the stomach lining.

Do not have unprotected sex or share needles. You can get an HPV infection by having sex with someone who is infected.

You can get hepatitis B, hepatitis C, or HIV infection from having unprotected sex or sharing needles with someone who is infected.

You may want to consider getting the vaccine that prevents hepatitis B infection. Health care workers and others who come into contact with other people's blood should ask their doctor about this vaccine.

If you think you may be at risk for HIV or hepatitis infection, ask your doctor about being tested. These infections may not cause symptoms, but blood tests can show whether the virus is present. If so, the doctor may suggest treatment. Also, the doctor can tell you how to avoid infecting other people.

If you have stomach problems, see a doctor. Infection with H. pylori can be detected and treated.

Certain Hormones

Doctors may recommend hormones (estrogen alone or estrogen along with progestin) to help control problems (such as hot flashes, vaginal dryness, and thinning bones) that may occur during menopause. However, studies show that menopausal hormone therapy can cause serious side effects. Hormones may increase the risk of breast cancer, heart attack, stroke, or blood clots.

A woman considering menopausal hormone therapy should discuss the possible risks and benefits with her doctor.

Diethylstilbestrol (DES), a form of estrogen, was given to some pregnant women in the United States between about 1940 and 1971. Women who took DES during pregnancy may have a slightly higher risk of developing breast cancer. Their daughters have an increased risk of developing a rare type of cancer of the cervix. The possible effects on their sons are under study.

Women who believe they took DES and daughters who may have been exposed to DES before birth should talk with their doctor about having checkups.

Family History of Cancer

Most cancers develop because of changes (mutations) in genes. A normal cell may become a cancer cell after a series of gene changes occur. Tobacco use, certain viruses, or other factors in a person's lifestyle or environment can cause such changes in certain types of cells.

Some gene changes that increase the risk of cancer are passed from parent to child. These changes are present at birth in all cells of the body.

It is uncommon for cancer to run in a family. However, certain types of cancer do occur more often in some families than in the rest of the population. For example, melanoma and cancers of the breast, ovary, prostate, and colon sometimes run in families. Several cases of the same cancer type in a family may be linked to inherited gene changes, which may increase the chance of developing cancers. However, environmental factors may also be involved. Most of the time, multiple cases of cancer in a family are just a matter of chance.

If you think you may have a pattern of a certain type of cancer in your family, you may want to talk to your doctor. Your doctor may suggest ways to try to reduce your risk of cancer. Your doctor also may suggest exams that can detect cancer early.

You may want to ask your doctor about genetic testing. These tests can check for certain inherited gene changes that increase the chance of developing cancer. But inheriting a gene change does not mean that you will definitely develop cancer. It means that you have an increased chance of developing the disease.

Alcohol

Having more than two drinks each day for many years may increase the chance of developing cancers of the mouth, throat, esophagus, larynx, liver, and breast. The risk increases with the amount of alcohol that a person drinks. For most of these cancers, the risk is higher for a drinker who uses tobacco.

Doctors advise people who drink to do so in moderation. Drinking in moderation means no more than one drink per day for women and no more than two drinks per day for men.

Poor Diet, Lack of Physical Activity, or Being Overweight

People who have a poor diet, do not have enough physical activity, or are overweight may be at increased risk of several types of cancer. For example, studies suggest that people whose diet is high in fat have an increased risk of cancers of the colon, uterus, and prostate. Lack of physical activity and being overweight are risk factors for cancers of the breast, colon, esophagus, kidney, and uterus.

Choose a diet rich in fruits and vegetables.

Having a healthy diet, being physically active, and maintaining a healthy weight may help reduce cancer risk. Doctors suggest the following:

- **Eat well:** A healthy diet includes plenty of foods that are high in fiber, vitamins, and minerals. This includes whole-grain breads and cereals and 5 to 9 servings of fruits and vegetables every day. Also, a healthy diet means limiting foods high in fat (such as butter, whole milk, fried foods, and red meat).

- **Be active and maintain a healthy weight:** Physical activity can help control your weight and reduce body fat. Most scientists agree that it is a good idea for an adult to have moderate physical activity (such as brisk walking) for at least 30 minutes on 5 or more days each week.

The Promise of Cancer Research

Researchers all over the world are looking for new and better ways to prevent, detect, diagnose, and treat cancer. They are learning more about what causes cancer. They are conducting many types of clinical trials.

A clinical trial is one of the final stages of a long and careful research process. The search for new treatments begins in the lab. If an approach seems promising in the lab, the next step is to see how the treatment affects cancer in animals and whether it has harmful effects. Of course, treatments that work well in the lab or in animals do not always work well in people. Clinical trials are needed to find out whether new approaches to cancer prevention, detection, diagnosis, and treatment are safe and effective.

Clinical trials contribute to knowledge and progress against cancer. Research already has led to many advances, and scientists continue to search for more effective approaches. Because of progress made through clinical trials, many people treated for cancer are living longer. Many of these cancer survivors also have a better quality of life compared to survivors in the past.

There are several types of clinical trials:

- **Prevention trials:** These studies look at whether certain substances (such as vitamins or drugs), diet changes, or lifestyle changes can lower the risk of cancer.

- **Screening trials:** These studies test methods of finding cancer before a person has any symptoms. Researchers study lab tests and imaging procedures that may detect specific types of cancer.

- **Treatment trials:** Treatment studies look at new treatments and new combinations of existing treatments. Examples include the study of drugs that kill cancer cells in new ways, new methods of surgery or radiation therapy, and new approaches such as vaccines.

- **Quality of life (supportive care) trials:** Scientists study ways to improve the comfort and quality of life of people with cancer. For example, doctors may study drugs that reduce the side effects of chemotherapy. Or they may explore ways to prevent weight loss or control pain.

People who join clinical trials may be among the first to benefit if a new approach turns out to be effective. And even if participants do not benefit directly, they still make an important contribution by helping doctors learn more about cancer and how to prevent, detect, and control it. Although clinical trials may pose some risks, researchers do all they can to protect their patients.

SECTION II B:

Cancer: Inside and Outside Environmental Factors

Cancer is a renegade system of growth inside the human body as already explained. The changes that must occur inside for cancer to flourish are genetic changes, but factors outside the body also play a role.

Humans do not exist in contaminant-free surroundings. Over a lifetime, a person's internal genetic makeup persistently interacts with external factors. Factors outside the body such as diet, smoking, alcohol use, hormone levels, or exposures to certain viruses and cancer-linked chemicals (carcinogens) over time may collectively conspire with internal genetic mutations to destabilize normal checks and balances on growth and maturation.

What Is the Environment?

When most people think of the word "environment," they think of forests, oceans, or mountains. In cancer research, however, scientists define the environment as everything outside the body that enters and interacts with it. This interaction is called an exposure. So, environmental exposures can include such factors as sunshine, radiation, hormones, viruses, bacteria, and chemicals in the air, water, food, and workplace, as well as lifestyle choices like cigarette smoking, excessive alcohol consumption (more than 2 drinks/day), an unhealthful diet, lack of exercise, or sexual behavior that increases one's exposure.

Researchers have estimated that as many as 2 in 3 cases of cancer (67 percent) are linked to some type of environmental factor, including use--or abuse--of tobacco, alcohol, and food, as well as exposures to radiation, infectious agents, and substances in the air, water, and soil.

Avoidable Environmental Factors

The good news is that the major environmental factors that are linked to cancer deaths can be modified, because most of them involve lifestyle choices. Almost one-third of all cancer deaths could be prevented by eliminating the use of tobacco products, for example, and making better dietary choices could prevent many more premature deaths from this disease. Our knowledge and certainty about diet is much less firm than it is for tobacco. Diets are very complex and we need to know what people ate in the past that impacted their cancer diagnoses today.

Influencing Rates and Risks

The environment *influences* cancer rates and risks. We can see this by comparing cancer rates in different countries, and how rates change when people move from one country to another.

For example, U.S.-born Japanese men have twice the rate of colon cancer as native-born Japanese men, and U.S.-born Japanese women have colon cancer rates 40 percent higher than their counterparts born in Japan. So scientists study what exposures or characteristics differ between Japanese immigrants and their descendants in the U.S. to better understand the environmental factors that may be influencing their colon cancer rates and risks.

Different Exposures, Different Rates and Risks

Certain types of exposures are linked to specific cancers. For example, exposure to asbestos is linked to lung cancer, and exposure to Benzedrine (a chemical found in some dyes) is linked to bladder cancer. Exposure to carcinogens from tobacco use is linked to several types of cancer, including cancers of the lung, bladder, mouth, lip, throat, voice box, and esophagus.

The Inside Matters: Random Gene Changes

Of course, environmental exposures by themselves do not cause cancer. Cancer is complex and involves many gene-gene interactions that occur inside you and are not well understood. For example, certain randomly occurring gene changes may be accumulating in your body's cells right now. And these same kinds of changes *may not be* occurring in your friends, your coworkers, or even your family members, even though all of you remain in a similar environment most of the time. Over your lifetime, random gene changes are passed along as your body cells grow and divide, so they accumulate. The unique patterns that evolve over time may make some people more likely than others to increase their risk for cancer after exposure to a particular chemical or after choosing a particular behavior.

The Inside Matters: Other Factors

You might wonder why some families are more cancer prone than others. In part, inheritance is involved in some of these cases as explained. This is because, at birth, some offspring unknowingly inherit gene changes that can make them more susceptible to cancer. But this explains only a very small percent of new cancer cases, no more than 5 percent.

Others factors that may change your cancer risk include having stronger or weaker immune systems, variations in detoxifying enzymes or repair genes, or differences in hormone levels.

Familial Rates and Risk: Those We Are Beginning To Understand

Rarely, several generations of the same family will develop the same type of cancer at rates much higher than those that occur in the population overall. Often, the family members are passing on mutated genes that impart a higher than average risk for developing this particular cancer. By studying the genetic profiles of these affected families, researchers are learning which genes are involved in cancer's development. Kidney cancer families are a good example of this. When scientists discovered the gene changes involved in the inherited form of renal cancer, they were able to use this information to better detect and diagnose sporadic or randomly occurring new cases of this cancer type. Only about 2 to 5 percent of cancers run in families this way.

Familial Rates and Risk: Those We Still Don't Understand

Some families will exhibit higher than average rates of a particular cancer, yet when scientists search their genomes, they are unable to find the usual genomic alterations suspected of increasing cancer risk. These cases seem to point to gaps in our understanding of the full set of mutations required for cancer's development. They also prompt researchers to probe deeper in search of possible environmental exposures suffered by the clan collectively.

Faulty Gene Repair Activities

Normally, if environmental exposures cause an unwanted molecule to bind to a gene, excision repair proteins rapidly remove that damaged area of the gene. Because the genes in the body that produce these repair proteins can themselves have mutations, people can differ from one to another in their gene repair activities. Unfortunately, genetic variations can make a person's gene repair activities less efficient or more error-prone than normal, and this faulty condition can be passed from generation to generation.

Hyperactive Detoxifying Activities

Other genes in the body produce detoxifying proteins that prepare toxic molecules for quick removal. Again, genetic variation in genes for detoxifying proteins can result in differences from one person to another in the ability to eliminate cancer-causing compounds. On the other hand, some genetic variation may actually produce hyperactive detoxifying gene activity. Then a person who possesses hyperactive detoxifying proteins may have some protection from harmful environmental exposures. Scientists believe, for example, that some persons inherit genes for hyperactive detoxifier proteins in lung tissues. This inheritance may partly explain why some smokers who refuse to give up the habit can still remain free of cancer. (For more information, please see *Genetic Variation*.)

Chance of Cancer? It Depends...

We know that some exposures increase the risk of cancer, but we don't know which specific combinations of environmental factors on the outside of the body combine with gene changes on the inside to lead to cancer. We don't know why two persons can have very similar environmental exposures, yet one gets cancer and the other does not. A number of individual factors are involved and there are complex relationships among them.

The individual chance that someone will develop cancer in response to a particular, single environmental exposure depends on how long and how often that person was exposed. It also depends on the person's:

- exposures to certain environmental factors (including diet, hormones)

- genetic makeup

- age and gender

Environmental Carcinogens: The "Nastiest" Lineup

Every two years, the Federal Government publishes a report on environmental exposures that have been linked to cancer. The most recent report included more than 220 substances. It helps to understand which of these exposures have the most impact on the general public.

As you consider these factors one at a time, it is important to remember that an individual accumulates a unique set of responses to his or her unique environment over a lifetime. Lengths and strengths of exposures will vary, and the person's genome itself will change.

Overweight and Exercise

Being overweight is an important lifestyle factor related to cancer risk. There are links between obesity and the risks of breast cancer (in older women), endometrial cancer, and cancers of the kidney, colon, and esophagus. Not being physically active increases the risk of colorectal and breast cancers.

Together, obesity and physical inactivity are linked to about 30 percent of the cases of colon, endometrial, kidney, and esophageal cancers, as well as 30 percent of breast cancers in older women.

Losing weight and exercising can help reduce your risk. Exercise at least 30 minutes a day, most days of the week. Exercise alone can decrease the risk of colon cancer and breast cancer. The goal should be for adults age 20 or older to keep their Body Mass Index (BMI) below 25. The BMI is a number that shows your body weight adjusted for your height.

Ultraviolet (UV) Radiation

Ultraviolet radiation--which comes from natural sunlight, sunlamps, or tanning beds--can lead to melanoma and other forms of skin cancer. While some sun exposure is good for health, excessive exposure during childhood seems a particularly important factor that increases skin cancer risk, and repeated exposure as an adult can increase risk as well.

Radon

This section explains the radon factor further than it was first introduced as a risk factor. Radon, a naturally occurring radioactive gas found at low levels in most soil, is produced in the soil when the element uranium starts to break down. The health effects of high radon levels were first seen in the increased cases of lung cancer found in underground uranium miners in the United States and around the world.

Radon gas seeps into cracks in the foundation of homes from surrounding soil; about 1 in 20 homes has elevated radon levels. Research estimates that about 20,000 lung cancer deaths every year may be linked to radon exposures in homes.

Check the radon levels in your home regularly. A ventilation system in your basement can dramatically reduce radon levels.

Diagnostic and Screening X-Rays

X-rays, mammograms, and radiation therapy all involve exposure to ionizing radiation. An X-ray of the chest exposes a patient to only a small amount of radiation-- about the same as one gets from two airplane flights across the United States.

Studies have not shown an elevated cancer risk associated with X-rays taken to diagnose a disease or condition. One exception to this is in children whose mothers received X-rays while pregnant: the children were found to have increased risks of leukemia and other types of cancers. Because of this finding, using X-rays to diagnose a condition in pregnant women are no longer recommended.

Talk with your doctor about the need for each X-ray that he or she suggests. Ask about shields to protect other parts of your body during an X-ray.

Radiation Therapy

Radiation to treat a condition--such as cancer or ringworm--is more likely to increase cancer risk. For example, people who receive radiation to treat conditions of the head and neck have an increased risk of thyroid cancer and of tumors of the head and neck.

Medications

Some chemotherapy drugs used to treat cancer may increase the risk of second cancers later in life. Drugs that suppress the immune system--used to treat some cancers as well as to prepare patients receiving organ transplants--also are associated with increased risk of cancer, particularly lymphoma.

On the other hand, new estrogen-blocking drugs called aromatize inhibitors can decrease the recurrence of breast cancer.

Any medication carries risks and benefits, so always check with a health professional before starting a new drug.

Solvents

Solvents are used in paint removers, grease removers, paint thinners, and dry cleaning. The solvents benzene, carbon tetrachloride, chloroform, and methylene chloride have been linked to human cancer.

The strongest evidence linking a solvent to cancer involves benzene, which is also found in cigarette smoke and gasoline. It increases the risk of leukemia.

If you must work with solvents, work outside or make sure the area is well ventilated.

Fiber and Dusts

Some fibers and dusts can increase the risk of lung-related cancers.

Asbestos is linked to increased risks of lung cancer and mesothelioma, a rare cancer of the lining of the lung and abdominal cavity. In the past, asbestos was widely used in construction, but its use has been restricted. However, workers employed in construction, electrical work, or carpentry may still be exposed through renovations or asbestos-removal projects.

Other fibers and dusts (including silica dust and wood dust) can increase the risks of cancers of the lung, nasal cavities, and sinuses.

Wear a well-fitting mask if your job exposes you to fine particles, fibers, or dust.

Dioxins

Dioxins are byproducts of paper bleaching, smelting, and waste incineration. They are widespread in the environment because they break down very slowly. They also accumulate in fat cells. Most of our exposure to dioxins comes from eating dairy products, fish, and meat.

Polycyclic Aromatic Hydrocarbons

These compounds (known as PAHs) come from the burning of carbon-based material. They are found in wood smoke, car exhaust, cigarette smoke, and charcoal-grilled foods. Sausages and roasted coffees may also contain PAHs. These compounds have been linked to increased risks of lung, skin, and urinary cancers.

Other Carcinogens: Metals

Some metals--including arsenic, beryllium, cadmium, chromium, lead, and nickel--have been associated with several types of cancer, including lung, kidney, brain, skin, and liver cancers.

Other Carcinogens: Vinyl Chloride

Vinyl chloride is used in the plastics industry and has been associated with lung cancer and with angiosarcomas (blood-vessel tumors) of the liver and brain. Most people are not routinely exposed to vinyl chloride unless they work in plastics manufacturing plants. People who live close to such plants also may be exposed through contaminated air.

Other Carcinogens: Benzedrine

Benzedrine has been known to be associated with cancer since the 1920s. It is used in the production of dyes for paper, textiles, and leather. Exposure to these dyed products is not hazardous, however.

Other Carcinogens: Aflatoxins

Aflatoxins are produced by certain types of fungi that grow on grains and peanuts. People can also be exposed to aflatoxins by eating meat or dairy products from animals that ate contaminated feed. Exposure to high levels of aflatoxins increases the risk of liver cancer. Peanuts are screened for aflatoxins in most countries, including the United States.

Identifying Cancer-Causing Substances

Americans commonly use more than 100,000 chemicals, and this doesn't take into account mixtures or combinations of chemicals. Plus, some chemicals are altered by the atmosphere, water, or incineration.

Scientists have been working for several decades to identify substances that cause cancer. They have three ways to do this: through human studies, animal studies, and laboratory experiments.

Human Studies

Human studies are the way to decide with the most certainty whether a substance causes cancer.

By following groups of people over time, researchers may be able to see whether certain exposures lead to cancer. They also compare a group of people who have been diagnosed with a type of cancer to another group of people without the disease. Sometimes the group with cancer has patterns of exposures very different from the patterns in the group without cancer.

Many environmental causes of cancer have first been noticed in the workplace, because people in certain occupations have higher exposures to some chemicals than do people in the general population.

Animal Studies

Rodents (mice and rats) are commonly used in studies of environmental causes of cancer. They have a relatively short lifespan (2 to 3 years), and their bodies' responses to known cancer causing chemicals are similar to a human response. Dietary studies in rodents are more difficult, however, due to differences in the digestive systems of rodents and humans.

In animal studies, the chemical exposures are usually at much higher levels than would be seen with human exposure. If an extremely high level of exposure does not lead to cancer, researchers reason that the chemical most likely does not cause cancer at lower levels either.

Laboratory Studies of Human Cells

Researchers study human cells in the laboratory to see whether certain chemicals might cause changes that could lead to cancer.

These studies are often done to see if animal studies--which take longer and are more complex-- are actually needed. If a chemical does not cause cancer in laboratory cells, animal studies usually aren't done.

Risk Assessment

How do scientists decide which exposures are high risk and which is low risk? Risk assessment involves three factors:

1. Potency: The potential of a given amount of a substance to cause cancer. Benzene, for example, is quite potent because even small amounts of it can increase cancer risk. Other compounds, such as chloroform, are less potent; they require higher exposures to increase the risk by the same degree.

2. Type of exposure: Whether the exposure is one-time (acute) or long-term (chronic), and whether it is unavoidable (in the workplace, for example, or in the air we breathe).

3. Dose response: A dose-response trend describes what happens to cancer risk as the level of exposure increases or decreases.

Occupational Cancer Risks

Certain occupations carry an increased cancer risk: these include painters; furniture makers; workers in the iron, steel, coal, and rubber industries; and workers involved in shoe manufacturing and repair.

Always use proper protective equipment when handling chemicals, and clean spills immediately.

Ask at your workplace about Material Safety Data Sheets, which contain information about hazardous substances.

The National Institute for Occupational Safety and Health (http:/www.cdc.gov/noish) can answer many of your questions.

Cancer Screening for Early Detection

Cancer screening tests help detect cancer at an early stage, which allows treatment to occur before the cancer spreads.

Get screened regularly for these cancers:

- **Colon/rectum:** Tests include the fecal occult blood test, sigmoidoscopy, and colonoscopy.

- **Breast:** The standard screening test is a mammogram, or X-ray of the breast tissue.

- **Cervix:** The standard screening test is the Pap smear.

Guidelines for when testing should begin and how often it should occur may be different for each person, so talk with your doctor about what's right for you.

Also talk with your health care provider about exposures at work and at home, and discuss whether your family or personal history may put you at risk for certain types of cancer. Your doctor may recommend other cancer screening tests as well.

Always Remember the Avoidable Risks

While it is always prudent to be aware of environmental exposures to carcinogens, one must also remember that the major environmental factors linked to cancer deaths can be avoided, because most of them involve behavior choices.

More than half of all cancer deaths could be prevented by eliminating the use of tobacco products, moderating the use of alcohol, and making better dietary choices.

My last word is that, Hope is on the way due to a myriad of factors. These include global research efforts backed by numerous global leaders and governments, as well as private corporations, such as President Barack Obama's signature health care reforms and its provision made for cancer research and general search for cure.

I wish you all the best and great quality of life.

(You can get more information on specific forms of Cancer and most current related research information at www.cancer.gov *: National Cancer Institute website)*

Appendix I: Helpful Diet

- Cabbage

- Chinese Cabbage

- Collard Green

- Dailcon

- Horseradish

- Kale

- Kohlrabi

- Mustard greens

- Arugula

- Beet greens

- Bok Choy

- Broccoli

- Brussels sprout

- Cauliflower

- Radish

- Rutabagas

- Swiss Chad

- Turnips

- Water cross

- Green Tea

- Flax seed

Appendix II: Some US Government funding for Cancer Research:

CENTERS FOR DISEASE CONTROL AND PREVENTION (CDC)

"The CDC leads the nation's efforts in cancer prevention and control. It conducts and supports research designed to better understand the factors that increase cancer risk and identify methods to prevent the disease. CDC state-based cancer programs provide vital resources for cancer monitoring and surveillance, breast and cervical cancer screening, state cancer control planning and implementation, and awareness initiatives targeting specific cancers."

CDC Federal Appropriations
FY2010-FY2012 (in millions)

	FY2010 Appropriation	FY2011 Appropriation	FY2012 Appropriation
CDC Cancer Programs			
Comprehensive Cancer Control Initiative	$20.69	$20.3	$20
National Cancer Registries Program	$51.24	$50.3	$50
National Breast & Cervical Cancer Early Detection Program	$214.85	$206	$206
Colorectal Cancer Screening, Education & Outreach	$44.53	$43	$43
Skin Cancer Prevention Programs	$2.19	$2.15	$2
Prostate Cancer Awareness Campaign	$13.64	$13.19	$13
Ovarian Cancer Control Initiative	$5.71	$4.91	$5
Geraldine Ferraro Blood Cancer Program	$4.67	$0	$0
Gynecologic Cancer & Education & Awareness (Johanna's Law)	$6.81	$0	$5

DEPARTMENT OF DEFENSE CONGRESSIONALLY DIRECTED MEDICAL RESEARCH PROGRAMS (CDMRP)

"In 1992, Congress established CDMRP at the Department of Defense (DoD). The peer-reviewed, biomedical research programs currently fund research in breast cancer, prostate and ovarian cancers. In the past, they have also supported research in other cancers, including chronic myelogenous leukemia and neurofibromatosis.

Because CDMRP is not considered part of the DoD's core mission, funding for DoD cancer research originates with Congress as part of the appropriations process, rather than in the president's budget. Consumer advocates and survivors play a primary role in setting priorities and influencing funding decisions."

DOD Federal Appropriations FY2010-FY2012 (in millions)

	FY2010	FY2011	FY2012
	Appropriation	Appropriation	Appropriation
Breast Cancer	$150	$150	$120
Ovarian Cancer	$19	$20	$16
Prostate Cancer	$80	$80	$80
Lung Cancer	N/A	$12.8	$10.2

NATIONAL CANCER INSTITUTE (NCI)

"NCI is the federal government's principal agency for cancer research and training. More than half of the NCI budget is allocated to research project grants that are awarded to scientists who work at local hospitals and universities throughout the country. More than 6,500 research grants are funded at more than 150 cancer centers and specialized research facilities located in 49 states."

NCI Federal Appropriations
FY2010-FY2012 (in millions)

	FY2010	FY2011	FY2012
	Appropriation	Appropriation	Appropriation
NCI	$5,103	$5,058	$5,081

Source: American Association for Cancer Research -
http://www.aacr.org/home/public--
media/science-policy--government-
affairs/resources-for-policymakers/federal-
cancer-research-funding.aspx

Appendix III: Affordable care act provisions advance fight against cancer.

PROVISION	SIGNIFICANCE FOR CANCER DISCOVERY AND CARE
CLINICAL TRIALS COVERAGE Prevents insurance companies from denying cancer patients participation in clinical trials or denying coverage of routine medical services clinical trial participants would otherwise be provided; covers all clinical trial stages for cancer and other life-threatening diseases. Implemented in 2010	The development of new ways to diagnose, prevent, and treat cancer depends upon a robust clinical trial system. Unfortunately, fewer than 5 percent of adults with cancer each year will participate in a clinical trial. This provision will remove a major barrier to participation and allow more patients to enroll.
COMPARATIVE EFFECTIVENESS RESEARCH Established an independent nonprofit center, the Patient Centered Outcomes Research Institute (PCORI), to conduct and oversee research that compares the clinical effectiveness of medical treatments. Research findings are prohibited from being construed as guidance for payment, coverage, or treatment. Appropriated funding began in FY 2010	By helping researchers to identify, and clinicians and patients to better predict which interventions will deliver the best treatment to the right patients, the results of CER studies can improve patient outcomes while improving overall healthcare value.
HEALTH DISPARITIES Elevated the National Center on Minority Health and Health Disparities to "institute" status within the NIH, giving it more authority to better coordinate and manage minority health and health disparities research. Implemented in 2010	Many minority and underserved population groups suffer disproportionately from cancer; multidisciplinary research is needed to uncover major factors in cancer disparities, such as genetics, lifestyle and behavior, to help reduce the unequal burden of cancer in the United States.
TRANSLATIONAL RESEARCH Created a new office within the NIH charged with speeding translation of basic scientific discoveries into treatments for patients. The Cures Acceleration Network (CAN) will provide grants of up to $15 million per year, per project, to both industry and academic research to speed translational research. $50 million authorized for FY 2011	Barriers between basic and clinical research make it difficult to translate new scientific discoveries to the clinic and patients – and back again to the laboratory. CAN promises to help overcome these barriers and speed more therapies to patients struggling with cancer and other diseases.
PREVENTION AND PUBLIC HEALTH Mandates $15 billion over 10 years for a Prevention and Public Health Fund that will support prevention and public health programs across the country, including for prevention research. Appropriated funding began in FY 2010	Nearly half of all cancers could be averted through preventative measures such as lifestyle changes and vaccines. This fund will support programs that target obesity, tobacco use, and other behaviors that put people at greater risk for cancer.
GENERIC BIOLOGIC DRUGS Authorizes the FDA to approve generic versions of biologic drugs and grant biologics manufacturers 12 years of exclusive use before generics can be developed. Implemented in 2010	By putting in place a framework to safely and accurately develop lower-cost therapies, it is anticipated that patients will benefit from the cost savings and exclusivity provisions will preserve incentives to innovators.
COVERAGE FOR TOBACCO CESSATION Requires that Medicaid cover tobacco cessation programs for pregnant women who are smokers. Implemented in 2010	Tobacco use and secondhand smoke pose serious health risks to mothers and their babies. Tobacco accounts for at least 30 percent of all cancer deaths and 87 percent of lung cancer deaths.
BREAST CANCER RESEARCH AND PREVENTION Directs the CDC to develop and implement a national education campaign about the threat breast cancer poses to young women; directs NIH to conduct research to develop and validate new screening tests and methods for prevention and early detection of breast cancer in young women. Implemented in 2010	Breast cancer is the leading cause of cancer deaths in women under the age of 40. Breast cancers found in younger women are generally more aggressive, are diagnosed at a later stage, and result in lower survival rates.

Source: American Association for Cancer
Research -
http://www.aacr.org/Uploads/DocumentRep
ository/LegAffairs/HCReform_Cancer_2010
.pdf

CITATIONS / REFERENCES

1. Richard L. Wahl, MD, Progress in Nuclear Medicine Imaging of Cancers, Primary Care Vol. 25, Number 2. June 1998

2. Roy van der Meel, William M. Gallagher, Sabrina Oliveira, Aisling E. O'Connor, Raymond M. Schiffelers and Annette T. Byrne, Recent Advances in Molecular Imaging Biomarkers in Cancer, Application of bench to bedside technologies, Drug Discover Today. Volume 15, Number 3 / 4. February 2010

3. Quantitative in Vivo functional imaging, Vol. 6 Supp 6, September 1999

4. Leonard Fass, Imaging and Cancer: A review, Molecular Oncology 2 (2008) 115-152.

5. National Cancer Institute website

6. National Cancer Institute, US National Institute of Health/www.cancer.gov, Cancer Trends, progress Report – 2009 / 2010 Update

7. National Cancer Institute website

8. S. Aslam Sohib, Dow – Mu Koh, Janet E. Husband, The role of Imaging in the Diagnosis, staging and management of Testicular Cancer, Genitourinary, Royal Marsden Hospital, Down Rd, Sutton, Surrey 10, 2007 accepted for revision Feb 4 2008

9. Michael S. Gee, PhD, Rasi Updhyay, BS, Henry Bergquist, BS, Herlen

Alencar, MD, Fred Reynolds, PhD, Marco Maricevish, MD, Ralph Weisslender MD, PhD, Lee Josephson, PhD and Umar Mahmood, MD, PhD, Human Breast Cancer, Tumor Models, Molecular Imaging of Drugs Susceptibility and Dosing during Her2/Neu-targeted Therapy 1, 1 From the Center for Molecular Imaging Research, Massachusetts General Hospital, and Harvard Medical School, Simches 8226, 185 Cambridge St Boston MA 02114

10. Wolfgang Stefan, Improving the quality of medical images, Arizona State University, Feb 4/ 2006.

11. Tilo Nieman, Thilo Kollmann, and Georg Bongartz, Diagnostic Performance of Low-Dose CT for

Detecting of Urolithiasis: A meta-analysis,DOT: 102214/AJR.07.3414, Revised Nov 12, 2007, accepted after revision Feb 23, 2008

12. Gregory A. Baxes, Digital Image Processing (Principles and applications, Publisher, John Willey & Sons , Inc, ISBN 0-471-00949-0 (paper)

13. Roy van der Meel, William M. Gallager, Sabrina Olivera, Aisling E. O'Connor, Raymond M. Schifelers and Annette T. Byrne, Recent advances in molecular imaging biomarker in Cancer: application of bench to bedside technologies, Drug Discovery Today-Volume 15, Numbers ¾- February 2010.

14. Prof. Jens Overgaard, Radiology and Oncology,(Molecular Imaging and

Radiation Oncology), Volume 94, supplement 1, March 2010

15. Sarah J. Nelson, PhD,* Edward Graves, PhD, Andrea Pirzkall, MD, Xiaojuan Li, MS, Antionette Antiniw Chan, MS, Daniel B. Vigneron, PhD, and Tracy R. McKnight, PhD, In Vivo Molecular Imaging for Planning Radiation Therapy of Gliomas: an Application of 1H MRSI, JOURNAL OF MAGNETIC RESONANCE IMAGING 16:464–476 (2002)

16. American Association for Cancer Research - http://www.aacr.org/home/public--media/science-policy--government-affairs/resources-for-policymakers/federal-cancer-research-funding.aspx

17. American Association for Cancer Research - http://www.aacr.org/Uploads/Docum entRepository/LegAffairs/HCReform _Cancer_2010.pdf

"Deux Lux Scientiae"